This Medical Appointments Tracker belongs to

_____

_____

Medical Appointments

Name	Date

Doctor	Hospital	Symptoms

Reason	Prescription	Notes

Lab and Test Results

Date	Test name	Results

Medical Appointments

Name	Date

Doctor	Hospital	Symptoms

Reason	Prescription	Notes

Lab and Test Results

Date	Test name	Results

Medical Appointments

Name	Date

Doctor	Hospital	Symptoms

Reason	Prescription	Notes

Lab and Test Results

Date	Test name	Results

Medical Appointments

Name	Date

Doctor	Hospital	Symptoms

Reason	Prescription	Notes

Lab and Test Results

Date	Test name	Results

Medical Appointments

Name	Date

Doctor	Hospital	Symptoms

Reason	Prescription	Notes

Lab and Test Results

Date	Test name	Results

Medical Appointments

Name	Date

Doctor	Hospital	Symptoms

Reason	Prescription	Notes

Lab and Test Results

Date	Test name	Results

Medical Appointments

Name	Date

Doctor	Hospital	Symptoms

Reason	Prescription	Notes

Lab and Test Results

Date	Test name	Results

Medical Appointments

Name	Date

Doctor	Hospital	Symptoms

Reason	Prescription	Notes

Lab and Test Results

Date	Test name	Results

Medical Appointments

Name	Date

Doctor	Hospital	Symptoms

Reason	Prescription	Notes

Lab and Test Results

Date	Test name	Results

Medical Appointments

Name	Date

Doctor	Hospital	Symptoms

Reason	Prescription	Notes

Lab and Test Results

Date	Test name	Results

Medical Appointments

Name	Date

Doctor	Hospital	Symptoms

Reason	Prescription	Notes

Lab and Test Results

Date	Test name	Results

Medical Appointments

Name	Date

Doctor	Hospital	Symptoms

Reason	Prescription	Notes

Lab and Test Results

Date	Test name	Results

Medical Appointments

Name	Date

Doctor	Hospital	Symptoms

Reason	Prescription	Notes

Lab and Test Results

Date	Test name	Results

Medical Appointments

Name	Date

Doctor	Hospital	Symptoms

Reason	Prescription	Notes

Lab and Test Results

Date	Test name	Results

Medical Appointments

Name	Date

Doctor	Hospital	Symptoms

Reason	Prescription	Notes

Lab and Test Results

Date	Test name	Results

Medical Appointments

Name	Date

Doctor	Hospital	Symptoms

Reason	Prescription	Notes

Lab and Test Results

Date	Test name	Results

Medical Appointments

Name	Date

Doctor	Hospital	Symptoms

Reason	Prescription	Notes

Lab and Test Results

Date	Test name	Results

Medical Appointments

Name	Date

Doctor	Hospital	Symptoms

Reason	Prescription	Notes

Lab and Test Results

Date	Test name	Results

Medical Appointments

Name	Date

Doctor	Hospital	Symptoms

Reason	Prescription	Notes

Lab and Test Results

Date	Test name	Results

Medical Appointments

Name	Date

Doctor	Hospital	Symptoms

Reason	Prescription	Notes

Lab and Test Results

Date	Test name	Results

Medical Appointments

Name	Date

Doctor	Hospital	Symptoms

Reason	Prescription	Notes

Lab and Test Results

Date	Test name	Results

Medical Appointments

Name	Date

Doctor	Hospital	Symptoms

Reason	Prescription	Notes

Lab and Test Results

Date	Test name	Results

Medical Appointments

Name	Date

Doctor	Hospital	Symptoms

Reason	Prescription	Notes

Lab and Test Results

Date	Test name	Results

Medical Appointments

Name	Date

Doctor	Hospital	Symptoms

Reason	Prescription	Notes

Lab and Test Results

Date	Test name	Results

Medical Appointments

Name	Date

Doctor	Hospital	Symptoms

Reason	Prescription	Notes

Lab and Test Results

Date	Test name	Results

Medical Appointments

Name	Date

Doctor	Hospital	Symptoms

Reason	Prescription	Notes

Lab and Test Results

Date	Test name	Results

Medical Appointments

Name	Date

Doctor	Hospital	Symptoms

Reason	Prescription	Notes

Lab and Test Results

Date	Test name	Results

Medical Appointments

Name	Date

Doctor	Hospital	Symptoms

Reason	Prescription	Notes

Lab and Test Results

Date	Test name	Results

Medical Appointments

Name	Date

Doctor	Hospital	Symptoms

Reason	Prescription	Notes

Lab and Test Results

Date	Test name	Results

Medical Appointments

Name	Date

Doctor	Hospital	Symptoms

Reason	Prescription	Notes

Lab and Test Results

Date	Test name	Results

Medical Appointments

Name	Date

Doctor	Hospital	Symptoms

Reason	Prescription	Notes

Lab and Test Results

Date	Test name	Results

Medical Appointments

Name	Date

Doctor	Hospital	Symptoms

Reason	Prescription	Notes

Lab and Test Results

Date	Test name	Results

Medical Appointments

Name	Date

Doctor	Hospital	Symptoms

Reason	Prescription	Notes

Lab and Test Results

Date	Test name	Results

Medical Appointments

Name	Date

Doctor	Hospital	Symptoms

Reason	Prescription	Notes

Lab and Test Results

Date	Test name	Results

Medical Appointments

Name	Date

Doctor	Hospital	Symptoms

Reason	Prescription	Notes

Lab and Test Results

Date	Test name	Results

Medical Appointments

Name	Date

Doctor	Hospital	Symptoms

Reason	Prescription	Notes

Lab and Test Results

Date	Test name	Results

Medical Appointments

Name	Date

Doctor	Hospital	Symptoms

Reason	Prescription	Notes

Lab and Test Results

Date	Test name	Results

Medical Appointments

Name	Date

Doctor	Hospital	Symptoms

Reason	Prescription	Notes

Lab and Test Results

Date	Test name	Results

Medical Appointments

Name	Date

Doctor	Hospital	Symptoms

Reason	Prescription	Notes

Lab and Test Results

Date	Test name	Results

Medical Appointments

Name	Date

Doctor	Hospital	Symptoms

Reason	Prescription	Notes

Lab and Test Results

Date	Test name	Results

Medical Appointments

Name	Date

Doctor	Hospital	Symptoms

Reason	Prescription	Notes

Lab and Test Results

Date	Test name	Results

Medical Appointments

Name	Date

Doctor	Hospital	Symptoms

Reason	Prescription	Notes

Lab and Test Results

Date	Test name	Results

Medical Appointments

Name	Date

Doctor	Hospital	Symptoms

Reason	Prescription	Notes

Lab and Test Results

Date	Test name	Results

Medical Appointments

Name	Date

Doctor	Hospital	Symptoms

Reason	Prescription	Notes

Lab and Test Results

Date	Test name	Results

Medical Appointments

Name	Date

Doctor	Hospital	Symptoms

Reason	Prescription	Notes

Lab and Test Results

Date	Test name	Results

Medical Appointments

Name	Date

Doctor	Hospital	Symptoms

Reason	Prescription	Notes

Lab and Test Results

Date	Test name	Results

Medical Appointments

Name	Date

Doctor	Hospital	Symptoms

Reason	Prescription	Notes

Lab and Test Results

Date	Test name	Results

Medical Appointments

Name	Date

Doctor	Hospital	Symptoms

Reason	Prescription	Notes

Lab and Test Results

Date	Test name	Results

Medical Appointments

Name	Date

Doctor	Hospital	Symptoms

Reason	Prescription	Notes

Lab and Test Results

Date	Test name	Results